Breast Cancer Lifesaver Blueprint

5 Known Facts About Breast Cancer

Dr. Glad Peterson

copyright©2022 By Dr. Glad Peterson
All publishing rights exclusively belong to Dr. Glad Peterson
 No part of this publication may be reproduced or transmitted in any form or by any means, electronic or mechanical, including photocopying, recording or by any information storage and retrieval system, without permission in writing from the publisher.

TABLE OF CONTENTS

Introduction.. 5

1. Most Common Disease................................ 10

2. Your Gene Can Play a Role 16

3. Men Are at Risk as Well ………..…............... 20

4. Malignant Bosom Bumps 24

5. There's No Age Limit 28

Introduction

When cells in your breast tissue begin to divide uncontrollably, forming a mass of tissue known as cancer, breast cancer can occur. You might remember feeling a bump on your bosom, noticing a change in the size of your bosom, or seeing changes in the skin on your bosoms. These are all signs of malignant growth in the bosom. Mammograms can help pinpoint early breast cancer.

We are all aware of the term "breast cancer" these days, which refers to a condition brought on by the abnormal growth of breast cells. According to research, women are more susceptible than men. It mostly affects the conduits or lobules of the breast, making it one of the most well-known female diseases studied. To avoid this terrible condition, every woman should take preventative measures, and having accurate information about its primary cause is unquestionably necessary. If you don't have it, grab it now by looking down.

Causes:

Despite the fact that the main factor that causes breast cancer in women is unknown at this time. However, there are a few things that increase your risk of being affected by the disease, such as maturing: Although reality maturing is one of the typical variables, it is difficult to accept. Your risk of contracting the disease increases with age as well.

Consumption of Liquor: Excessive alcohol consumption also increases your risk, so you should limit your intake to avoid it.

Tissue of the Breasts: The condition could also be caused by having thick bosom tissue. It might aid in the growth of the infection-causing cells.

The early fetus cycle: Women who start having periods before the age of 12 are more likely than other women to experience confusion.

Late labor or never being pregnant: Some women who, for whatever reason, have their first child at a later age are more likely to develop the bosom disease because of one problem or another. Additionally, it affects women who are unable to think clearly.

Family or Past History: If you have a malignant growth in one of your bosoms, you probably also have one on the opposite side. Additionally, if anyone in your family has had it in the past, this may double the likelihood that you will develop breast cancer.

These are a few of the factors that raise your likelihood of developing breast cancer. In addition, assuming you are the person with the condition, rather than allowing yourself to feel at ease, proceed to seek legitimate treatment that increases your chances of recovery. The problem can be fixed with a variety of treatments, such as surgery, radiotherapy, chemotherapy, hormone or endocrine therapy, and so on. Always seek treatment for your bosom malignant growth according to your current condition.

In the United States and the United Kingdom today, breast cancer is a major concern for all individuals. Due to the development of breast malignant growth mindfulness, people are very aware of the risks. Some women are actively seeking screenings to prevent malignant growth from developing and are adopting healthier lifestyles to do so. People who are certain they have the disease can choose from a variety of options for malignant growth treatment. Integrative treatments like chelation and ozone can be found in a variety of elective disease treatment centers.

The following resources will be helpful to you if you are interested in learning more about this disease to protect yourself.

1. Most Common Disease

Did you know that breast cancer is the second most common malignant growth found in women in the United States? It is also the second most common cause of illness-related death among women of all races and identities. Unfortunately, many people are unaware of the risks, which are made worse by poor lifestyle choices. You can speak with a doctor at an elective disease treatment center if you were found to have this kind of malignant growth. The person in question will teach you about diet and lifestyle changes that are likely to help your condition.

It is anticipated that bosom disease will account for 32% of female malignant growth cases and 14% of the expected 282,500 female disease deaths in 2017. One in eight women will develop a malignant growth in their bosom.

While there is no definitive method for preventing breast disease and many risk factors cannot be changed, monitoring the following most common risk factors can assist you in managing those that are within your control.

• Bosom disease is more prevalent in females than in males by a large margin.

• Age: Two-thirds of women with obtrusive breast malignancy are over 55 years old.

• Family history If your mother, sister, or girl has had breast cancer, your odds are even higher. If two members of your immediate family have it, your risk is much higher. The screening guidelines change slightly depending on family ancestry, so talk to your primary care physician about what's best for you.

1.It's an Epidemic This dangerous disease is spreading, especially among women in the United States and the United Kingdom. According to the numbers, there will be 230,000 new cases of obtrusive breast disease in the United States this year. About 40,000 of these women will die from the disease. It is heartening to learn that over 2.5 million people in the United States have overcome breast cancer. This demonstrates that early detection is crucial to surviving the disease. Over the past few years, the number of people who die from this kind of illness has gone down. The best signs of progress are coming from women under the age of 50.

With an estimated 1.4 million new cases analyzed annually, bosom disease is the most well-known malignancy affecting women overall. The created world holds the most elevated occurrence; Regardless, frequency rates are always rising in various parts of the world. Between the years 2002 and 2020, the prevalence of breast cancer and mortality are expected to rise by half, with the greatest increase occurring in non-industrial nations.

To explain this rate increase, a few hypotheses have been put forth, the majority of which focus on the shifts in way of life that occur as countries become more westernized. For instance, the cervical cancer is the most common malignant growth among women in India; However, when these women move to the

United States, bosom disease becomes the most widely recognized malignancy.

Comparative changes have been observed in various studies assessing the frequency of breast malignant growth in foreigners from low-asset or developing nations. Within nations, urbanization grows at the same rate; For instance, breast cancer rates in China's metropolitan vaults have increased by 20-30% over the past ten years. This shift is connected to improved screening methods, diet, and lifestyle changes.

Bosom disease risk factors like weight, early menarche, and diminished or late childbearing are becoming more prevalent as regions become more evolved. As these numbers continue to rise, it is essential to keep in mind the limited resources and other social beliefs in this area, as well as the significance of devising a novel and compelling strategy for reducing the developing breast disease problem.

2. Your Gene Can Play a Role

Your risk of developing the disease doubles if you have a close family member who has breast cancer, such as a mother, child, or sister. In any case, it's also important to remember that over 85% of patients have no family history of the disease. Sadly, many women over 40 who do not have a family history of the disease avoid annual screenings.

About 4% to 10% of cases of bosom disease are thought to be inherited, which means that they are simply the result of changes in quality (transformations) passed down from one parent to another.

BRCAs 1 and 2:An acquired change in BRCA1 or BRCA2 quality is the most well-known cause of innate bosom disease. These characteristics aid in the production of proteins that repair damaged DNA in typical cells. The development of strange cells, which can lead to disease, can be sparked by altered adaptations of these qualities.

• You are more likely to develop a malignant growth in your bosom if you have inherited a modified copy of one quality from a parent.

• A woman with a BRCA1 or BRCA2 quality mutation has a 75% chance of developing breast cancer by the age of 80. The number of other relatives who have had bosom disease also affects this chance. It rises in the event that more relatives are affected.)

• Women who have one of these changes are more likely to be diagnosed with bosom malignant growth and disease in both of their bosoms at a younger age.

• Women who have one of these quality changes are also more likely to develop ovarian cancer and other types of tumors. Additionally, men with one of these quality changes are more likely to develop breast and other malignant growths.

3. Men Are at Risk as Well

Many people are surprised by this because it's not often discussed in the media. In any case, it is certain that men can encourage this kind of malignant growth. It is estimated that there will be 2,300 new obtrusive cases among men in 2022. The disease is expected to kill approximately 450 people. There are two out of every 1,500 chances that this will be fostered by a man. Despite the small number, men should not dismiss breast cancer as a possibility. Bosom disease can affect men, despite the fact that it is uncommon. Find out about male bosom disease side effects and factors that could increase your odds.

Although men can develop breast cancer, breast cancer is more common in women. In the United States, approximately one man is found to have one of the 100 identified bosom diseases.

- Intrusive ductal carcinoma is the most common type of benign growth in the male genital area. The disease cells originate in the conduits and later spread to various parts of the abdominal tissue outside of the channels. Malignant growth cells that are visible can also spread to other parts of the body, or metastasize.

• Lobular carcinoma that is visible. Malignant growth cells begin in the lobules and eventually spread to nearby bosom tissues from there. Additionally, these intrusive disease cells have the ability to spread throughout the body.

• Ductal carcinoma in situ (DCIS) is a disease of the breast that has the potential to initiate obtrusive breast malignant growth. The disease cells are only in the coating of the channels and have not spread to other bodily tissues.

Bosom tissue is present in everyone. The majority of men's breast tissue is behind the areola. Women have significantly more breast tissue than men do, and breast cancer grows at a much faster rate. Regardless, malignant growths can occur in male bosom tissue.

Male malignancy is exceptionally rare. Every year, around 150 men over the age of

50 in Australia are found to have a malignant growth in their bosom. The number of Australian men diagnosed with breast cancer each year is probably going to rise steadily as our population gets older. As a result, providing affected men and their families with information and support becomes increasingly important.

4. Malignant Bosom Bumps

Malignant growth in the bosom has the same side effects on men as it does on women, including the following:

- ✓ a change in the state of the bosom or areola;
- ✓ a release from the areola; an excruciating region;
- ✓ enlarged lymph hubs in the armpit region;
- ✓ a bosom irregularity;
- ✓ thickening of the bosom tissue;
- ✓ dimpling of the skin of the bosom.

A lot of women do get lumps in their bosoms, but these bumps aren't harmful. This suggests that they pose no threat to you. Blisters, blood clumps from an injury, benign cancers like fibroadenomas, mastitis, knobs, or scars are examples of these. Malignant growth has not been linked to any of these. Despite the fact that any cell-framed knot may be referred to as a growth in reality. Not all growths pose a threat or are harmful.75% of the bosom protrusions biopsied are benign (noncarcinogenic). The most common benign bump-producing conditions in the body are listed below.

As we have seen, the majority of irregularities in the abdomen are benign, non-destructive cancers or sores. They will not attack surrounding tissue, even if careful expulsion is required to prevent them from disrupting normal body capability; They do not pose a threat. However, dangerous breast cancers will continue to grow, attack, and destroy adjacent normal tissue if they are not detected and treated early. By a process known as metastasis, disease cells will split away from the cancer and spread to different parts of the body through the lymphatic system and circulatory system if they are left unchecked. Bosom malignant growth is dangerous at this stage, and in the early, confined stage, the chances of fixing it are much lower (roughly one-half).

Although areola emissions, changes in the appearance of the areola, areola tenderness, or dimpling or puckering of the skin may initially indicate the presence of some breast diseases, the majority of harmful cancers first manifest as single, hard knots or thickenings that are frequently, but not always, easy. These harmful bumps, which typically originate from the mammary organs or pipes, typically appear in the upper, external quadrant of the bosom, stretching into the armpit, where the tissue is thicker than elsewhere. (Approximately 50%)

The areola, lower out quadrant, and lower internal quadrant account for 18 percent, 11 percent, and 6 percent, respectively, of bosom diseases. Any change in size, shape, surface, or areola that occurs in one bosom may be more dangerous than if it occurs simultaneously in both similarly situated bosoms. Make the change known right away.

27

5. There's No Age Limit

It's feasible for both the youthful and old to have breast disease. Notwithstanding, its chances happening increases as you become older. As per the American Malignant growth Society, the chances of getting this illness at 20 years of age is 1 out of 1,750. And at 30 years of age, this increments to 1 out of 230, then, at that point, 1 of every 69 at 40 years of age and 1 out of 29 at 60 years of age. When you're 70, your gamble increments to 1 out of 27. The general lifetime risk for bosom disease is 1 out of 9.

It is vital that you know that breast cancer disease happens when cells in the bosom start to develop and duplicate unusually than normal. These changes can happen because of lifestyle choices, food or gene. Changes in DNA can make typical bosom cells become unusual.

The specific motivation behind why typical cells transform into dangerous cells is indistinct, yet specialists know that chemicals, ecological elements, and hereditary qualities each assume a part.

Breast screening is an approach to distinguishing breast disease, frequently at a beginning phase. It includes X-beams called mammograms.

This direction helps you know more about breas screening assuming that you are up to 70years or over and what you are qualified for.

In the event that you are above 71 or over, we don't consequently welcome you for bosom screening. In any case, you really do reserve the option to free screening like clockwork assuming you inquire. You should simply telephone or keep in touch with your neighborhood bosom screening unit to make an arrangement.

The number of ladies under 40 getting analyses of metastatic bosom disease is expanding. The movement to metastasis in bosom disease is more likely Trusted Source in juvenile and young ladies than in more seasoned ladies who have a determination of beginning phase bosom malignant growth.

Metastatic bosom disease implies that the malignant growth has progressed to organize

4. It has moved past the bosom tissue into different region of the body, like the bones or the cerebrum.

Endurance rates are lower for malignant growth that has metastasized to different pieces of the body.

As indicated by the American Disease Society, the 5-year endurance rate for ladies with bosom malignant growth that has spread to different pieces of the body is 28 percent Trusted Hotspot for all ages.

Among each age, juveniles and young ladies have lower bosom disease endurance rates than more seasoned ladies. The further developed the disease, the poorer Trusted Source the viewpoint in this gathering.

www.ingramcontent.com/pod-product-compliance
Lightning Source LLC
Chambersburg PA
CBHW050326220526
45465CB00005B/2146